Love Yourself Slimmer

The Energetic Approach to Releasing Weight

Caroline Nixon

ISBN-13: 9798619899597
ISBN-10: 1477123456

Cover design by: Art Painter
Library of Congress Control Number: 2018675309
Printed in the United States of America

CONTENTS

DEDICATION

This book is dedicated to those who have struggled with their weight for years or maybe even their whole life (maybe even many lifetimes). This is for you if you are so freaking tired and basically just done with all the yo-yo dieting bull. You are through beating yourself up and berating yourself constantly for your weight and your body.

This book is your light at the end of the tunnel; your lighthouse beacon that there is so much hope and love available for you. Are you ready to rediscover love for yourself and your body (and begin releasing weight because you want to feel amazing in your body)? Let's do this thing!! I got you! Together we rise, we shine and we kick booty cause that is how we roll.

FOREWORD

This book has been years in the making. My passion and purpose in this life is, and has always been, to help people love themselves. So simple, and yet how many of us simply do not love ourselves very much? We can spend our whole life berating ourselves and our bodies. We mask our emotions with food, (alcohol, shopping, decorating, redecorating, over exercising, sexual addiction) and so much more. I have been there for sure.

I believe with all of my heart that when you can come into a place of deep self love, you can move mountains. You can reach any goal you set, including releasing weight. It becomes much easier in fact, because you become your own best cheerleader for your goals. How amazing is that?

I believe that each of us are powerful creators, and we sometimes forget that we are which then causes all kinds of emotional, mental, physical and spiritual upheavals for us. Every moment is our chance to course correct and love ourselves for who we are right at this moment in time.

You are holding a book in your hands right now that will challenge you to think and feel differently about your body, your soul, your powerful self, everything. This weight loss book is like no other (and there are so many weight loss books on the market). This book is different because it points out and brings light to all

aspects of your body weight issue; not just the physical stuff (diet and exercise).

This book goes deeper into the real reasons you are holding onto extra weight. It also will help you pinpoint where you need to investigate further into your own life to uncover your root cause of your weight gain (or inability to release those pounds). But even further than that, you will learn (or re-learn) how to love YOU more!

What you are about to embark on is what I help my clients with all the time. I am giving you the farm as they say, because I really want you to not only release your extra weight so that you can feel amazing in your body, but I want you to love the heck out of yourself so that you can create the life of your dreams with way more ease and joy.

What you need to know before you even begin reading this book, is that I am an intuitive energy healer (for over 20 years). I read the energy of the body (and everything is energy). I can move energy that is stuck, release old patterns and programs, and I can show you where you are limiting yourself. That is my true passion and calling.

So be warned that you will hear me speak of all things "out there" and "woo", but really and truly they are just the truth of who you

are and who you can become more of if you allow your heart and soul to receive it. Also I am not a doctor. I do not diagnose, claim to cure, prescribe or any of those "doctor-y type" words. I work with energy (and everything is energy). Always seek professional medical advice as you need. Do not stop taking any medications without first consulting with your medical practitioner. Advocate for your highest and best health and wellness though. Find a doctor that is open minded and who will listen to you and your unique needs.

With all of that out the way, I cannot wait for you to begin digging into this book and begin seeing how your body, mind and soul shift into a healthier, happier you. There are a lot of exercises here for you to explore. Do them. Do not just skip by them telling yourself that you will do them later. They are important part of your self exploration. Use them. Play with them and you will discover so much about yourself in the process.

With so much love,
Caroline Nixon
March 2020

CONTENTS

INTRODUCTION

If you have ever carried extra weight on your body, you know how hard it can be. How something as simple as picking out your clothes in the morning becomes an ordeal, where you are choosing clothes to hide your butt or your stomach rolls. You know. You know how much time and energy you can spend throughout the day thinking about how you look; feeling heavy and frumpy and judging yourself harshly for every perceived flaw.

It sucks, doesn't it? I know. I lived this way for too long. What a waste of precious energy worrying about my body which I chose by the way, then proceeded to berate for years and years. When you think of it like that, it seems almost ridiculous (not even almost-it is ridiculous). Worrying, fretting, obsessing, chastising, shaming and guilt-ing my body is what I did and who I was quietly, privately in the comfort of my own head for years!! I was never one of those people who really talked about my weight, my ass, my belly. Nope, I was a more suffer (and obsess) in silence type of gal. Cause if I didn't address it, it would be like it wasn't real, right? And what is even crazier is I was not really overweight as a teenager; I just thought I was. Talk about crazy making!!

Having these preconceived notions of what beauty was and having a sister who was the opposite of me physically speaking, really messed with my head for a long time. Again I chose this before I came into this body on this planet (in my view we choose before we incarnate). We are a soul, in a body, having a human experience after all. The irony is not lost on me there. Divine comedy for sure. It still sucked.

Back to being overweight. So we can all agree it sucks, even if you are only 10 pounds all the way up to 100 pounds (or more) heavier than you wish you were. I think it is safe to say we all want to feel comfortable in our bodies, sexy even or perhaps just attractive if sexy feels like too much of a stretch. There are so many factors to being overweight. There are so many ways to lose weight as well. The weight loss industry is big business. I don't personally feel there is any ONE way to lose weight.   I believe there are a lot of components to address and then there is YOUR particular way. I am so excited to share my knowledge and experience with you, so that you can begin to love and trust your awesome body and release your extra weight once and for all.

I have created this book, which is like no other experience out there. It combines all of the different aspects of weight issues. This is not a diet or exercise program. If you are looking for a meal plan or exercise regime, this is not the book for you. This is a deep dive into YOU; your beliefs, your blocks, your past unresolved emotional upsets, your subconscious programming, your physical and spiritual practices, that you will begin exploring while having compassion and love for your journey and experiences.

And we will have some fun too. Deeply transformational healing that is fun? YES!! People are so serious, are they not? Healing can be fun, light and playful. In fact that is very high vibin. I don't feel like we need to suffer any longer to be able to reclaim our health (and our slimmer bodies). We can release all that "stuff" and lose weight with way more ease, flow and joy than we ever dreamed possible.

So if you are tired of the weight loss yo-yo dieting, and are open minded, I know this book will help you not only reduce your weight but love yourself so much more. That is the key after all to lasting body changes; love. At the root of ALL that ails you is your subconscious programming and unresolved experiences, which can then lead to inner resistance, unworthiness issues and lack of self love (and dis-ease in the body).

Are you ready to get started on this life changing journey? Let's get this party started then. In the first few chapters I will begin to lay out all of the many, many causes of why you might be overweight and unable to lose the weight you want to lose. You see, most of the time we only focus on the physical stuff, like diet and exercise. That is just the tip of the iceberg my friends. I would even go so far to say that the food you eat and the movement you perform (or lack of movement) are mere symptoms of what is really going on deep inside your subconscious.

There are other areas of yourself which need to be examined with loving eyes in order to truly heal and release your extra weight for good. You gotta look at your beliefs, thoughts and programming (the mental stuff). You need to address (not re-live however) all of your past emotional upsets that are unexpressed and literally festering in your body. And then there is the spiritual side of you that you need to explore.

As I said earlier, you are a soul, in a body, having a human experience. Your soul is eternal and wise and has experienced many, many, many lifetimes here on Earth (and dare I say other places as well). Remember how I said earlier to have an open mind? Now is the time because I will be discussing past lives in this book.

This book is not just a book that you read though. Nope. This book can also be considered a workbook, a journal, a place to gather your thoughts as you deepen your connection with yourself; as you love yourself more. There are worksheets for you to fill out, journal prompts, positive affirmations (and afformations-more later on this).

This book is meant to be your road map to inner freedom and deep self love and forgiveness. Oh and there are website links sprinkled throughout with recording energy healings for you to access and listen to for even more profound results. Excited yet? I am. I am ready to witness your transformation and success! I hold that intention for you. I know you can release and heal your connection with your body, mind and soul, so that you can finally, with way more ease and joy, release the extra body weight that you have been carrying for years from a place of love.

SOME PRE-WORK EXPLORATION

Before we get into the meat and potatoes of this book, I want you to think about a few things. Use the space below to write your thoughts down. Be honest with yourself here, but also be loving. You cannot change, shift or heal what you are not willing to acknowledge.

Right now my body feels...

When I lose the weight, I will feel...

Can you look for ways to feel that way right now?

List 5 things (or more) that you have been afraid to do (or too self conscious to do) because of your weight and how you feel about your body?

1.

2.

3.

4.

5.

"You are never too old to set another goal or dream a new dream."

-C.S. Lewis

CHAPTER 1

What does love have to do with it?

You may be wondering why I chose to call this book, *Love Yourself Slimmer*. Why not call it something more marketable like, *How to lose 10 pounds in 10 days?* Surely that would sell more copies. And while that might in fact be true, that is not how I work with people. I don't believe that is how weight loss should be approached. Holding onto extra body weight, struggling with foods and strict exercise regimes does not treat the root cause of your weight issues (at least not in my view).

Everything is energy, and oftentimes with weight issues we are just not loving our bodies too much. We might even dip into hate, loathing, disgust when we think about our bodies and ourselves. And society (the collective consciousness) tells us that in order to lose weight we gotta go on a diet and use our conscious mind (about 5-10% of you) to tap into our willpower to lose the weight. They say we gotta power through and restrict what we eat.

Pushing through your cravings, counting calories, depriving yourself, exercising for hours, etc. are recommended for success. And you can absolutely lose weight if you go this route. You can lose a lot of weight actually. People do it all the time. They usually, however gain all that weight back (and more) once they "fall off the wagon" and begin eating again, or when they have a stressful day and just grab the first thing in the pantry.

Does this way of losing weight actually heal the root cause of the weight issues though? I think it treats the symptoms but not necessarily the real reason behind the extra weight.

Does this way of losing weight help you love your body more? I suppose if you love how you look after the weight loss, then it does. But what happens if you gain that weight back? Do you hate your body all over again? How many cycles of that have you been through in your life?

Here's a scenario I want to lay out for you. Really imagine what I am about to say and breathe it in for a moment. What if you never lose your extra weight? What if you spend your entire life at the weight you are right now? No changes, no matter what you do or how much you punish your body. Would you spend the rest of your life hating yourself and being miserable? Would you be able to just stop all of your body shaming and accept (and really just love) all of you? Your answer will be very telling for you.

If you can heal your thoughts, beliefs, programming around dieting and foods, you can literally change how you view foods and eating. Your cravings for those less healthful foods magically diminish and your body is able to naturally regulate and re-balance itself (aka release weight). Everything is energy. Fact. Thoughts are things. Fact. What you focus your attention on, grows. Read that again because it is so important. If you are constantly thinking that you need to lose weight or if you are constantly thinking how fat you look or gross you feel, THAT is your focus and the Universe brings you more of that energy to experience (because that is where your attention is). And all that inner conflict and negativity creates disharmony in your body (aka inflammation), which then leads to more weight gain, lower immune function, sluggish body systems and disharmony. Know that a huge part of your weight struggles are because of your beliefs about it, and we will getting into those beliefs soon.

When you begin to love yourself for who you are right now and where you are right now, your body begins to relax and unwind from all of that chaotic energy and negative self talk. You begin to take better care of yourself and get your needs met in healthy ways that feel really good. You are able to put yourself first, fill your own cup and say "no" to people as needed. Doesn't that sound amazing? It is totally possible for you. Getting into the energy of love (which is so high vibin) will help your body self regulate, heal, re-balance itself while feeling so much more peaceful. As a result of the inner work your are doing, your outer world (aka your body) will begin to shed those pounds almost magically and with so much more ease and flow.

Try this simple exercise right now to get into the energy of self love. Get a little mirror out or go into your bathroom and just look into your eyes for a moment. And as you are looking into your eyes, I want you to smile. Notice how your eyes begin to light up. Then tell yourself (via your eyes) that you love you. You can also just wrap your arms around yourself right now and give yourself a little hug. This is a baby step to that you can do anytime to get into the energy of appreciation, gratitude and love.

In the next section, I am going to be asking you some powerful questions. Take your time and be honest with yourself. You will begin discovering some of your own beliefs around your body and releasing weight.

Journal Time

I cannot express how important journaling is to heal your relationship with yourself and your body. Let's get started below with a few journal prompts. Take your time and allow whatever arises to just be. If you are afraid that someone will read your journal entries, you can either journal on a separate piece of paper and rip it up or burn it when you are through. Or you can type it on your computer and simply delete it afterwards. There is no right way to journal. Do not allow fear to keep you from digging deep into your feelings here. So much insight can be brought to light from journaling. Give it a try and see what comes up for you.

How long have you struggled with your weight?

Why do you want to release weight?

____

____

____

____

____

____

____

Why do you think/feel you are not able to release weight (or keep it off)?

____

____

____

____

____

____

____

____

____

Let's play a game!
Rate your weight loss struggles from 1-10
(1 being your biggest struggle)

*I don't know where to even begin losing weight.

*Time management (I am too freaking busy.)

*Putting myself first (Everybody comes before me.)

*Healthy boundaries (I don't know how to say "no" to people.)

*Stress eating (I eat when I am sad and happy.)

*Not moving my body enough. (Exercise sucks.)

*My hormones are out of whack.

*My emotions are all over the place. (I am up, down and every which way.)

*I don't know.

*All of it!!

Once you have rated your struggles from 1-10, just take a moment and let your answers sink in.

Sometimes you don't even know something is an issue for you until you see it right in front of your face. This little game is just to make you aware of your struggles at the beginning of this book. It is not yet another way to berate yourself!! That is not helpful, at all.

Body part exercise

Imagine or visualize a part of your body that you don't like or feel good about (your booty, your tummy rolls, your chin, your arms, your thighs, etc.). Just pick one for now.

With that one part of your body in mind, take a few slow, deep breaths and feel into, get a good sense of or visualize that one part, fully and completely. Pretend here. Imagine. You can even touch it.

Now ask that one part of your body that you do not like, what message it would like to give you right now. Again, be open to receive a message. Pretend that body part is talking to you. You are not crazy.

Just notice what you notice. You may see, hear, feel the message. Be open to how you receive your intuitive information.

Once you have received your message, ask that one body part what you can do to help it right now. Ask what it needs to feel better; to feel loved.

Again, just notice what you notice. There is no right or wrong answer here.

Now thank that one body part.

Tell that one body part how much you appreciate it. Tell it how grateful you are for it and all that it does for you on a daily basis. Tell that body body how sorry you are for ignoring it, berating it, hating it. And if you can, tell that one body part that you are going to begin loving it so much more.

This can be a very powerful healing exercise, if you allow it to be. I encourage you to give this a try. Be open, receptive and present with whatever comes up for you. You may be shocked at the messages your body has for you.

"How can I love myself
more today?"

-Me

CHAPTER 2

What is energy healing?

Nowadays people are becoming more and more familiar with the term, "energy healing". But what is it? It sounds so far out. One must first become aware that everything is energy. We are all energy, frequency, vibration, pure and simple. This is a scientific fact. Everything has a vibration, a frequency; the chair, the plants, each cell in your body. We appear solid, but when you break it down, down, down, we are pure potential energy.

Within our bodies, we have energy centers (chakras), meridian lines (energetic highways) and around our bodies we have what are referred to as "energy bodies", the energy that makes up our aura.

And know that your energy can get stuck, just like a pipe can get clogged. When your energy gets clogged up and blocked, you can feel tired, have aches and pains, mood swings, weight gain, and if your energy remains stuck for a long time dis-ease can set in. Ultimately disease is the physical representation of a lot of stuck, inflamed energies that have remained unresolved for a long time.

When we are feeling good, we are vibrating at a higher frequency. And when we are not feeling so well, our vibes are lower. This is a constant thing for us. We are never just one vibration or frequency. We move up and down as life and experiences occur and how we respond to and process these experiences.

Many things can clog up your energy, but when you begin to break it down, the biggest things that muck up your energy are unresolved emotions, past traumas and your beliefs (your programming). Essentially we are a big 'ol bag of emotions and beliefs in a human suit.

Energy healing therefore is simply working with energy to balance and harmonize the body, mind and soul. Energy healing unsticks, unclogs your energy (and therefore your body). Energy healing lovingly reminds you of your connection to Source, God, the Universe and that we are all connected to the all because we are all things (big, deep statement right there so read it again). It brings you back to love, self love, love of all.

There are so many different energy healing modalities available today. Too many in fact to list here. Know that not all energy healing modalities will resonate with you. You are unique and divine. Your needs are unique to you. Some energy healing modalities you will be drawn to explore, and I invite you to explore away. I have studied many different modalities in these past 20 years. Some I still use with my clients today, and some I have simply let go of because they no longer resonate for me.

When thinking about weight issues and energy healing, know that when you are able to pull up and clear all of that negative, limiting thinking and programs that you have been subconsciously been plugged into for so long, your body is able to re-balance, recalibrate and come into a healthier weight for you.

We will be going into this topic a lot more in later chapters, so keep on reading. I love using energy healing with my weight loss clients. If you are open to it, it can really help you begin to unravel so many beliefs and un-truths about yourself that are literally keeping you from releasing weight.

10 ways I can add more self care into my week!

1.

2.

3.

4.

5.

6.

7.

8.

9.

10.

CHAPTER 3

Why are you overweight?

So let me ask you a question. Your answer will help you begin to uncover your beliefs and programming. Be sure to check out the journal prompts in the previous pages as well. Take a deep breath as you answer the following questions honestly and with love and compassion for yourself.

Why are you overweight? Why do you think you are overweight? Why do you struggle with your weight? I will say that about right now, most people (usually women) I have spoken with and worked with say something like they don't exercise enough, they eat too much, their hormones are out of whack, etc. And while to some extent those answers may be true, I believe you need to dig a little deeper. Remember I said earlier that there are so many causes to weight gain and struggling to release weight. So many.

One of the first things I want to bring light to are your beliefs. Essentially you are just a big bag of beliefs and programming in a body suit. What you believe (whether it is true or not is irrelevant), becomes your experience. Read that again and let that sink in. If you believe that you have to eat only lettuce and run 10 miles a day to lose weight, then that is what it will take for you to see results. Your subconscious mind (where all your beliefs and programming are stored) does not know the difference between what is real and what is imagined, true or false. Your conscious mind is not running the show in your life; your subconscious mind is.

So if growing up, you were raised by parents who had certain ideas about weight, what it takes to be a healthy weight (or anything really), you as a young child would have soaked all that information into your subconscious mind even if it was total bull crap (which let's face it, most of it is). Breathe. Sometimes it is quite a shocker to realize that you have believed lies and untruths about yourself and what it really takes to live a life in a body you love. We have been programmed by our parents, families, society, the collective consciousness (you know, Muggles) to believe a lot of malarkey. It is no wonder we grow up and struggle with so much and are so unhappy.

The good news is that now that you know that your beliefs can and do dictate what you experience in your life, you can begin to examine what you believe and decide whether or not if you still want to. You can shift your beliefs thereby changing your life (hallelujah).

So let me ask you another question to keep the ball rolling. Be really honest with yourself right now. Do you believe that you can release weight? If your answer is "no", it will be way more challenging for you to have success with any program, healing, book. If you answer, "yes, but" those are the beliefs you will want to begin digging into. These dieting beliefs are ingrained very deeply within us. If we have lived on this planet, we have been literally soaking in soooo much garbage about dieting, losing weight, foods, all the things around what it means to be attractive. Let me just remind you that in other times (ie other lifetimes long ago), someone who carried a little bit more weight was considered wealthy, healthy and beautiful. Never allow current trends to affect your love of self. You are beautiful!

The most important thing for you to do right now is find out what you believe about losing weight. We will be diving into this more in chapter 5, but you can go ahead and start thinking about what you think, believe and feel you need to, have to, should do to lose weight. Make a list for yourself. "In order to lose weight, I have to..."

The next three chapters will dive deeper into all the many causes of why releasing weight can be challenging. Keep reading and discover some of the contributing causes you have been experiencing with your weight.

Journal Time

Why am I excited to release weight?

____

____

____

____

____

____

Why does losing weight scare me?

____

____

____

____

____

____

Am I ready to release my extra weight now?

____

____

____

"Once you replace negative thoughts with positive thoughts, you will start having positive results".

-Willie Nelson

CHAPTER 4

The physical causes of being overweight

This chapter will explain some of the biggest physical causes we often think of when we talk about losing weight. By the end of this chapter your perspective on solely focusing on the physical causes will be very different (I hope). What do you think of when you think about why you cannot lose weight? Everyone automatically thinks of diet and exercise, right?

Well, let me tell you, diets suck. They focus on restricting certain foods and they put you in "lack" mentality. Saying to yourself that you can't have this food or that food or that certain foods are "bad", causes all sorts of inner turmoil; a pushing and pulling for control. It literally sets up a battleground within your body, mind and soul.

Diets love to categorize foods as good and bad. Diets give food power; power over you. Then comes along different aspects of yourself (aka your shadow sides) like, "the rebel", "the victim", "the saboteur", "the martyr" to wreak even more havoc in your life.   These shadow sides of you (remember that you are made up of all things) pop up to show you where you still have some healing to do. If this interests you (and it is fascinating) do an internet search and explore away.

What happens when you tell yourself that you cannot have that chocolate cake? You will either use your willpower to resist the urge for the cake, or you will begin to crave it even more, right? Or maybe your rebellious self steps forward and says, "You can't tell me what to eat!"

If you start demonizing certain foods as being wrong, knowing that everything is energy and has a vibration (as I already discussed), then what do you think happens if you actually "cave in" and eat those demonized foods?

Guilt, shame, resentment, hatred, loathing is what happens. If you feel any of those emotions while (or after) you eat those demonized foods, you are literally spoon feeding that energy vibration into your body; your cells. What do you think THAT will do to your health and well-being (and weight loss efforts)? Well, nothing good I can promise you that. It lowers your vibration. And you feel bad about yourself once again.

Your belief about a certain food is so powerful. If you believe that a food is bad or wrong, then it will not be healthy for your body (because you believe that). Food is food. Food can heal and nourish, as well as weaken and deprive.

Now do not misunderstand me, I am not a huge fan of just eating "junky foods" with no real nutrients and tons of chemicals. However, if I choose to eat dessert, I just eat the dessert. I bless the heck out it (and sometimes I do some energy healing on it), and I simply enjoy the dessert. There is no guilt or shame. I do not worry about the calories or fat content. I eat it for the pleasure of it, and then I move on. And because I am in the moment and loving the thing I am eating, I am literally bringing all that positive energy into my body too. Bonus, right?

Can you see the difference? Would you rather deprive yourself of all foods, eat the foods and feel terrible about it or just enjoy the piece of cake (or whatever)? I know which one I would choose.

So I highly recommend ditching the dieting mindset. The goal here is to come into peace and harmony with all foods; not into a battleground. Energy healing can really help with this by the way. Check out the recording I made for you over at www.carolinenixon.net under "shop".

We do need to chat a bit more about food though. In good conscience I cannot and do not tell my clients to eat chemically laden, non-food, foods. There is no energy there, no real nutrition and it leaves your body craving (because of all the preservatives, additives and chemicals) more and more. It is just fillers, chemicals and toxins. The frequency of these non-foods is very low in general.

Eating a lot of these junky foods does not nourish your body. They are not able to. Sure your belly may get full, but your body has to work a heck of a lot harder to process them. And all those chemicals can really mess with your body systems. And you can set yourself up to keep craving them due to all the addictive chemicals they contain.

Remember when I said earlier that demonizing foods can cause all sorts of inner resistance (and ultimately health struggles)? It is true. While I do not personally consume much in the way of "junk" food, I do not beat myself up if I do decide to eat something less than optimal. There is no guilt or shame at my party. If I choose to eat something that is not so high vibin, I bless it (I may even run some healing on it), and then I just enjoy it.

I have found the more energy healing I do with my own body, and the more I nourish my body with whole, home cooked meals, the less I desire the junky foods. Sometimes if I begin to crave a certain food, I will stop right there and just check in with myself. Did I just get triggered by something or someone? Am I upset about something? Am I yearning for a feeling? Am I simply bored? Just doing that quick 30 second check in helps me release any craving I might be having. But again, since I do not demonize foods, I can also just eat that food (most likely I would have to go to the store since I don't buy those junkier foods) and move on.

Another thing you can do especially if your body is used to eating a lot of these non-foods, is to begin weaning yourself off of them slowly. Some folks like to complete clean out their cabinets and start fresh. If this is you, then go for it. I have found that a lot of people need a more gentle approach though if they want lasting changes to become the new normal. I suggest cutting back gradually, so your body does not go into a huge detox crisis. Ultimately it is up to you what you eat, but I promise you that your body will feel so much better when you nourish it with fresh, whole foods.

If you are used to dieting all of this may seem foreign to you. Most weight loss programs are so focused on foods. They dictate that you have to eat a certain way. There are so many different diet plans out there, and they all seem to contradict each other which can feel super confusing.

In my private practice, I am able to intuitively tune into my clients to help them decipher which foods are better suited for them. I bring in energy healing to help release the blocks, beliefs, programming and resistance so they can come into harmony and balance with all foods, themselves and their bodies. In time I find that they are able to let go of the struggle and embrace a more inclusive, holistic approach to nourishing their body.

△△△

Another physical cause of being overweight is exercise, or lack of movement. Again there are so many ways to work out; almost as many options at there are diets. And don't all of these fitness professional have the answer using their system? Of course. Over the years I have purchased so many different workout DVDS and downloadable programs. They are great dust collectors. I would try them a few times before giving up because they were either way too hard for me to do or I was bored. Can you relate? How many DVDs do you have collecting dust in your home? I have also joined many gyms over the years as well. I have learned after several years and a lot of monetary investments that I prefer to work out alone in my garage. I have what I need, and I have no excuse because my garage is right there within a few steps. But it is important to know how you prefer to work out. Maybe a group exercise class motivates you or walking with a friends floats your boat.

Personally I feel that building more movement into your day is vital and not just to lose weight. Your body needs movement for optimal health. Your joints need the lubrication, your body needs movement to lower your stress hormones, your lymphatic needs movement for the release of toxins and maintaining a healthy immune system, your nervous system needs movement to reduce stress.

When I exercise I focus on feeling strong and flexible. I even visualize myself strong and flexible as I work out. For me it is not about burning calories but about being really present in my body and feeling my muscles work as they lengthen and strengthen.

My intention is always to add more movement all throughout my day. I walk my dog several times a day. I dance in the kitchen as I prepare meals. I work out most mornings in my garage (typically strength training type exercises). I get up from my desk and walk around or stretch every hour or so (this is no problem since I drink so much water and need to go to the bathroom a lot). I also like to change up my workouts, so that I can challenge my body and different muscle groups.

If you do the same 'ol exercises day after day, your body gets used to it and is no longer challenged (which essentially defeats the purpose of exercising). Mix it up every so often. Make your exercise routine a lesson in mindfulness as well.

I practiced tae kwon do for years (I have my 2nd. degree black belt actually). One of the things I loved about taking a martial arts class was how different each workout was. My body was always challenged (and sore). I also had to concentrate a lot on my balance with my kicks and on remembering the forms. There was no zoning out like you can on a treadmill. If I lost my focus, I would fall over or whack myself in the head with a nunchucks (I did this a lot).

If you don't exercise or haven't in some time, go slow. Be gentle with your body. The easiest exercise to begin with is walking. Just go outside and walk. Honor your limits. You can also incorporate some stretching into your day. There are a million resources available online for you to choose from. The important thing to remember is to move your body more, be mindful with your movement and visualize yourself getting stronger, leaner, more flexible, etc. Always be sure to check with your medical provider before beginning any new workout regime.

△△△

Yet another physical cause of weight issues can be an underlying or diagnosed medical condition. You may have had an injury and needed to rest for a while, so then you began to notice some weight gain from lack of movement, eating more out of boredom etc. There are some physical issues like thyroid imbalances, blood sugar imbalances and moving into different phases of life that can cause the body to put on extra weight. These can also make it more challenging to release the weight as well.

I am not going to dispute the above because I know a lot of people who have experienced this type of weight gain. However, if you recall that everything is energy (I say this a lot if you haven't noticed), and your beliefs dictate your experiences, you realize that physical issues are just the symptoms of what is truly going on at the root (subconscious programming, unresolved emotional upsets and inner resistance). By the time your body physically manifests an illness or condition, it has been in your energy field for a while. Your physical body is the last stop on the train ride. I don't say this to blame you if this is your experience, but to gently remind you that all physical symptoms have an emotional root.

Sometimes the very medications you are prescribed can have an affect on your weight. If that is the case, I would personally do energy healing on the medication, I would also dig into why I am in need of the medication (ie look into the diagnosis more), but I would also check in with my doctor to see why this is happening and what else can be done to help alleviate the weight gain (that hopefully does not involve another pill).

△△△

We live in a world full of toxins. The foods we eat are genetically modified, full of pesticide residues, food additives, preservatives, colorings and more. The air we breathe is polluted (and most of us do not breathe properly anyway). We are inundated with electromagnetic fields (EMFs). We use harsh chemicals to "clean" our homes. The personal care products we use are full of chemicals. We work in places with fluorescent lighting and we avoid the sun at all costs. The pots and pans we use release toxins into the air (and into our food) and the microwaves we use destroy the nutrients and can leech plastic into our food. The impact of all of these toxins is huge. It is no wonder we are sick and overweight.

Have no fear though, for there are so many ways we can decrease our toxic load, thereby helping our bodies detox and move into harmony (and release weight).

First off, simply open your windows if the weather allows. The air in most homes (and cars) is stale and more polluted than the air outside. Change your air filters frequently as well. Using essential oils in your home can greatly enhance your overall health. I will be diving into the art of Aromatherapy and how it can support you in releasing weight in Chapter 9.

Use natural cleaners and personal products that are free of harsh chemicals. We are super lucky to live in a day and age where so many amazing natural products are available. Hop on your computer and search for natural cleaning products. You will be amazed at the choices available to you. Check out some of my rec-ommendations in the "stuff to check out" section at the end of the book.

A few more tips to help you reduce your toxic load so that your body can run more optimally (and release extra weight) include using less (or no) plastics. Drink out of a glass water bottle (or stainless steel). Use glass containers instead of plastic ones. There is a direct correlation between plastic use and hormonal disruptions. If your hormones are out of balance, so will your weight be. Never heat up food in a plastic container unless you want to ingest micro plastic bits. Look this up; it's a thing.

Reduce your exposure to EMFs by putting down your phone. Don't stare at any screen all day long. Get outside more. Soak up some vitamin D by being in the sun a bit more. There are all sorts of EMF cancelling devices you can find online. Check them out, and see what your options are for lower your exposure to

EMFs. And why not start a garden to grow some of your own food? Growing food is an amazing experience that gets you in touch with nature in a new way, and the food just tastes better.

△△△

There are a couple more physical causes to poor health in general (and weight struggles) that I want to address, as these are so easy to remedy (and they are either free or super cheap). Stop reading right now and take a slow, deep breath in through your nose and out through your mouth. Notice that I did not tell you to take a short, fast, shallow breath, yet this is exactly how most people breathe all day long especially when under stress (and everyone seems to be so stressed out). Most folks only breathe at about 1/3 of their lung capacity actually. We need air to live, and breathing is the way by which air comes in. The breath is what keeps our bodies alive through oxygen.

Deep breathing relaxes the mind, oxygenates the blood and regulates the autonomic nervous system. Shallow breathing deprives the cells, organs and glands of much needed oxygen. Lack of oxygen starves the brain, nervous system, adrenals, pituitary gland, kidneys, gallbladder, spleen, liver, diaphragm, colon (basically every part of your body). Shallow breathing is a response to being stressed out, and if you are stressed out all the time then chances are good that you are not breathing deeply and oxygenating your cells.

Proper deep breathing brings you into a more relaxed state of mind (more mindful, more present, more peace). It can alter your consciousness, affect your emotional health and it helps to clean your lymphathic system (your body's detox system).

When you are stressed out and not breathing deep enough, you may not make the best food choices. You may turn to food and booze to de-stress when you could just stop and take some deep breaths and bring yourself back to center.

There are tons of cool breathing exercises that you can learn. I like to breathe in through my nose to a count of 5 (or higher), then I hold it for a count of 5 (or more), then I release the breath through my mouth for a count of 5 (or more). This type of breathing will really bring you into the now moment. It is meditative and feels amazing.

I think you get the picture; breathe deeply often. Make deep breathing part of your day by either sitting in quiet contemplation/meditation or by taking a break every so often during your day to just breathe. Breathing deeply at stop lights can help curb any road rage you may be feeling too.

Now let's move on. Let me ask you a question, how's your sleep? Do you get enough sleep? Is it quality sleep? Do you fall asleep quickly and then wake up in the middle of the night wide awake? Do you toss and turn all night? Maybe you have trouble getting to sleep.

Getting enough quality sleep is so important for your overall health and wellbeing because when you sleep, your body repairs itself including boosting your immune system and toxins are able to be released. If you are not sleeping well, you just are not able to function optimally. You may lean on caffeine and sugar to get you through your day only to find that you cannot sleep at night. It can be a vicious cycle, and it can add extra weight to your body.

Signs of being sleep deprived can include: lowered immunity, daytime drowsiness, mood swings, high stress, lowered memory, having coordination issues and feeling disoriented or spaced out. Also studies have shown that when you do not get enough restful sleep your body actually produces more hunger hormones (ghrelin), which makes you hungrier so then you begin eat more as a result of not getting enough zzzzz's.

A couple of tips to help you get a good night's sleep are to limit your caffeine, especially in the afternoon, go to bed at the same time each night (it trains your body that it is time to rest), don't watch tv right before bed (it can stimulate you), drink herbal tea to wind down, take a hot bath, do some light stretching, journal to get out your day so you are not obsessing over an event that occurred and looking into taking some supplements. These are just a few of the many ways you can ensure you are able to fall asleep and stay asleep all night long. Just to let you know, drinking that glass or three of wine nightly might give you a feeling of being relaxed, but alcohol can in fact mess with your sleep cycle. Just keeping it real.

And lastly I would like to touch on hydration. Did you know that approximately 75% of the human body is water? Water is the regulator of all of your body's functions. All of your organs, muscles and bones contain water.

Do you drink enough water? I think that most folks are slightly to significantly dehydrated. Once you feel thirsty, you are already getting dehydrated. If your body's water level drops by just 2% you will begin to feel tired. If it drops by 10% you may see health issues arise. You may be wondering what water actually does for your body. A lot! Water improves oxygen delivery to your cells, it transports nutrients all throughout your body, it hydrates your cells, it moistens oxygen for easier breathing, it cushions your bones and joints, it absorbs shock to your organs and joints, it regulates your body temperature, it removes waste products and toxins, prevents your tissues from sticking together, lubricates your joints, improves cell to cell communication, maintains normal electrical properties in your cells and it empowers your body's natural healing processes. Thirsty yet?

Research has shown that being dehydrated renders your immune system less effective. Chronic dehydration contributes to so many health issues such as arthritis, asthma, colitis, depression, diabetes, ulcers, gastritis, heartburn, headaches, high blood pressure, high cholesterol levels, low back pain, neck pain, osteoporosis, kidney stones and more. If you struggle with any of the above, make sure you are drinking enough good quality water. And sorry, not sorry but caffeinated drinks and alcohol do not count. They actually dehydrate you.

If you find that you are wanting to eat or you get a craving, try drinking a glass of water first. Sometimes you are not really hungry at all. You are just needing water.

As you can tell, there are many physical causes and contributing factors to being overweight. This is but a tip of the iceberg however. Continue reading and learn mental, emotional and spiritual causes to your weight struggles and of course how to begin shifting them into more balance and love.

Tips & Tricks to help you!

*Do not wait until you are starving to eat or go grocery shopping

*Make a meal plan for the week (or month)

*Do not buy "junk" foods (your emotional trigger foods)

*Eat out less/Cook more

*Focus on eating nutrient dense foods

*Chew your food really well

*Drink less with meals (it dilutes your digestive juices)

*Notice how you feel during and after your meals

*Brush your teeth between meals or anytime you feel like snacking

*Eat off of smaller plates

*Build movement into your day (small bursts)

*Drink water with lemon to help your body detox

*Drink less alcohol and caffeine (makes you dehydrated and tired)

Journal Time

How has being overweight limited you?

____

____

____

____

____

____

How has being overweight served you?

____

____

Food Journal

For 5 days (yes, I said 5 days) I want you to write down every darn thing you eat (and drink). I know this is a bit of a pain. Knowing what you are putting into your mouth will help you, I promise. This is NOT about calories! This is not about judging your food choices. This is about you becoming really aware of what you are ingesting. You cannot change what you are not even aware of, right?

And as I mentioned earlier, your beliefs about food and eating can (and do) cause all sorts of inner resistance within your mind and body. Where there is resistance of any kind, there is disharmony which leads to inflammation, which leads ultimately to bloating, gas, pain, extra weight and in some cases dis-ease.

There is no judgment here. If you are not super honest with what you are eating, you won't be able to shift anything. I have included a simple chart for you to use if you desire. This is for your eyes only. At the end of the 5 days, take a look at your diet. Be kind with yourself. Knowing is the greatest first steps to making changes (with love and compassion of course).

Breakfast:

____

____

____

Lunch:

____

____

____

Dinner:

____

____

____

Snacks:

____

____

---

10 ways I can add more nutrition into my week.

1.

2.

3.

4.

5.

6.

7.

8.

9.

10.

10 ways I can add more movement into my week.

1.

2.

3.

4.

5.

6.

7.

8.

9.

10.

CHAPTER 5

The mental & emotional causes of being overweight

You are essentially a big bag of beliefs in a human suit. As stated earlier in the book, your subconscious mind runs the show in your life. As a result, your beliefs (mostly in your subconscious) ultimately dictate the experiences you have. So if you believe that losing weight is hard, sucks, is impossible, then guess what? It will be for you.

In this chapter, I want to talk about some of the biggest mental and emotional causes for weight issues. You may resonate with a lot of these or only a few. That is okay. With all things in this book (and in life itself), take what you like and leave the rest.

Let's face it, food is a big deal in our world. We celebrate with food. We reward ourselves with food. Teachers do this all the time in their classrooms. We console ourselves with food. We use food. Personally I love eating. Eating is a total pleasure. One of the perks I would say to being in a body. It becomes a problem when we use food to meet our emotional needs or when we try to escape from our lives. We, as a society, do this with food, alcohol and drugs all the time.

If you are running for a bag of chips, a chocolate cake or a bottle of booze at the end of the day because you had a rough, stressful day, then you might want to stop and take a look at that. Is it unconscious? Do you really want that thing, or has it just become an unhealthy habit or even an addiction? There is no judgement here. Be honest with yourself, but be loving and forgiving as well.

A lot of folks stuff down their feelings with food, because for whatever reason they are afraid to say that thing they really need to say to that person (a partner, friend, family member, co-worker, boss). Do you do this? If so, I suggest getting really real with yourself here. Write in your journal. If you don't feel like you can speak up directly to the person you have an issue with, then write them a letter. You do not have to send it. You can write it all out and then burn it or throw it away. The important thing is to not let your emotional upsets fester (and fester they will if you do not express them).

I mentioned earlier that your thoughts and beliefs about losing weight can literally stop you from actually losing weight. At the end of this chapter, I have included a really long list of limiting beliefs that I have found a lot of folks are plugged into (in their subconscious). We pick up these limiting beliefs as kids (or before) from our parents, families, society, the news, social media, etc. Because we are such little sponges as kids, we just soak it all up even if it is not true (and it is usually not true).

If you belief that you have to eat a certain way, do certain exercises, not eat this, not do that, etc, that will be your experience. It sounds so simple, but your beliefs are so powerful. Maybe it is time to examine some of your own beliefs about how hard it is to lose weight (hopefully you are already thinking about these). These will be the blocks to your success that you need to work with (don't worry I will help you later in the book).

Some people hold onto extra weight as a result of sexual trauma. I wish this was not such a huge issue in our world, but sadly it is. So many are victims of sexual abuse and trauma. When something like this happens, we can literally put on weight for what we feel is protection. We think that if we are overweight, no one will attack or abuse us. We try to become invisible to predators. Of course this is not consciously done. It is subconscious (90% of our beliefs are).

We may even block out traumatic events that occurred when we were younger because they were too painful. This happens so often. If this is resonating for you, I would advise speaking with a therapist who specializes in this type of work. Energy healing can absolutely help, but I feel it is important to work with someone who is trained in this type of issue specifically.

Sometimes we gain weight because are just stressed out from life, tired, in jobs we hate, we stay with partners we have out grown, we are stuck in the past (the good 'ol days) or we are living in the future (worry of what may come) and we are generally not feeling super passionate or fulfilled in our life. Mid-life crisis anyone? There seems to come a point in people's lives where they begin to question their life choices. Stereotypically speaking, this is when men start working out, ditch their wives and buy a sports car. I am joking a little, but you get the point.

And when you are stressed out all the time, your adrenal glands can get super taxed and tired. When that happens your hormones can get out of balance, and the stress hormone, cortisol, can actually make you crave fatty foods. When you can work on lowering your overall stress levels, your hormones can begin to rebalance, helping your body's weight to balance out as well.

Sometimes too, we can begin reflecting on our life and wake up one morning wondering what our life purpose is, why we are here, and realize that we aren't all that happy and we need to make some changes. This is sometimes referred to as the dark night of the soul (or mid life crisis although it can happen at any age).

We question everything. This can be a really good thing as long as you are courageous enough to actually make new choices and change what needs to be changed (and only you can do that). You can't just have ah-ha moments and not actually change anything in your life. If nothing changes, nothing changes, right?

When you stay in a job you know you need to leave, stay in a marriage that frankly sucks, bite your tongue so you don't upset someone, people please, have no healthy boundaries, you can feel bad about yourself, feel depressed, lose your zest for life, and you can turn to food and booze (and shopping and sex) to console yourself. Then you berate yourself for gaining weight and not being able to lose weight. You can even get sick because of all this emotional baggage you are pretending doesn't exist. This becomes a crappy way to exist.

There is another way. You can free yourself from all of this emotional pain. I will show you how in the coming chapters. You only need to be brave enough to look at where you have made choices that are not in your highest and best good. The good news is that you are the powerful creator in your life and you can always, always, always course correct by making a new choice and taking a new action. How awesome is that?

△△△

Exercise to get to the root

I asked you this question earlier in the book, but I want to take it a step further so that you can begin to heal. This is an advanced exercise. Go at it with an open mind, knowing and setting the intention that all that is revealed is in your highest and best good.

The question was, **"I am not able to release weight because..."**

Think about that for a moment. Your answers to that question are your beliefs and not necessarily the root cause of your weight issues. Remember that your weight issues are a symptom of something deeper that is going on within (physical, mental, emotional and spiritual causes). Close your eyes and take a deep breath. And I want you to connect with your Higher self, your most wise YOU; your soul self. Just say, "Higher self, Higher self, Higher self, I connect with you now."

Allow yourself to remain open and follow the energy through time and space as you ask your Higher self to show you the root cause of your particular weight struggles This may either be back in time through this life or before (in a past life) where the seed was planted for you to struggle with your weight. Notice what you see, sense, feel, feel. Use all of your senses for this exercise. Do not judge what comes up. Just witness it. Can you see yourself (or another you in a different time)? How old are you? What do you look like? Be open to all that arises here.

Does this person (you) have a message for you? Spend some time with this person (this other you) and find out, ask, watch, witness what was going on in that time that planted the seed to your current weight issues. Ask this person what they need to heal this struggle once and for all. Ask your Higher self and your spirit guide team for assistance with this.

Next, visualize that the person you are speaking with is completely healed and free of the weight struggle. See them smiling and happy. Ask them if they need anything further at this time. Thank them while you say out loud, "I mark this experience downloaded, complete, healed and fully integrated now." And take this a step further and say out loud, "I now step onto my highest and best timeline for optimal health and my perfect body weight. Thank you. It is done."

By now, you should be feeling pretty darn good. If this does not feel complete, you can always do the exercise again. When the root cause is healed and marked as complete, the body begins to automatically come into harmony and balance.

Limiting Beliefs to pull from your energetic self

Below I have listed a whole bunch of outdated, lower vibrational and not super helpful beliefs that you might be plugged into. Remember these beliefs that are stored in your subconscious mind have been taught by family, the society you live in and potentially past lifetimes. It is vital that these beliefs be pulled and replaced with higher vibrational truths. Think of this exercise like upgrading your computer hard drive with new software and getting rid of any computer glitches or malware.

How do you pull these beliefs you may be wondering? You can write down the ones that you resonate most with, and then journal on them. You can spend a bit of time digging into where you picked these up, who you learned them from, and then you can imagine them being released from your body, mind and soul.

You can also use energy healing to help energetically pull them from your subconscious. I have recorded an energy healing for you over at www.caroline-nixon.net (click the "shop" button) which energetically pulls all of these beliefs for you. They are pulled out of your cells, your chakras, meridians, energy bodies, ancestry line and more. This work is deep and sacred, and you will feel so much lighter afterwards. Not all of these statements will resonate with you, but these are the most common ones I see with clients. You may have some come up that are not on this list as well.

*I don't know why I am overweight.

*I have tried everything and nothing works for me.

*I have seen, doctors, therapists, nutritionists, healers and no one can help me.

*I don't think anything will work for me.

*Nothing works.

*Other people have success, but I do not.

*I feel so frustrated with my body.

*I feel so frustrated with my weight.

*I will always be overweight.

*I have to starve myself, restrict my diet, never eat carbs, fast for days and days to lose weight.

*I gain weight easily.

*I look like my mom/dad.

*It runs in my family.

*I have bad genes.

*I just look at carbs and gain weight.

*I have to/should give up gluten, dairy, meat, fat, sugar to lose weight.

*It is too hard to lose weight.

*Food is my enemy.

*Strict diets are the only way to lose weight.

*I have to exercise for hours daily to lose weight.

*I am just lazy.

*I should exercise more.

*I hate my body.

*I hate how I look.

*I beat myself up about my body.

*I am a fat slob.

*I am useless, stupid, a loser, unworthy.

*My body is gross.

*My body has failed me.

*My body is ugly.

*My weight is too much.

*I have lost all hope.

*I am disappointed in myself and my body.

*I feel heavy, frumpy and sluggish most of the time.

*I hate shopping for clothes.

*I look terrible in clothes.

*I hate seeing my body in the mirror.

*I am so self conscious about how I look.

*I am not sexy.

*I don't feel sexy.

*Nobody desires me.

*I am resolved to just be this way.

*I eat for comfort.

*I am insecure.

*I have tried and tried and cannot lose weight.

*I don't believe in myself.

*My past diets did not work.

*I need extra weight to keep me safe.

*I have to be heavy to be grounded.

*I am overweight because I take on other people's energy.

*I am a psychic sponge.

*It is not safe for me to lose weight.

*If I lose weight people will see me and that is not safe; it is scary.

*I eat the wrong foods.

*I eat too much.

*Food makes me sick.

*Gluten is toxic.

*Sugar is toxic.

*Meat is toxic.

*Dairy is toxic.

*I hate sugar, wheat, gluten, dairy, meat, fat and it hates me.

*Grains are toxic.

*Milk is toxic.

*Cheese is toxic.

*I only crave junk foods.

*I have no control over what I eat.

*My cravings are out of control.

*I am out of control.

*My life is out of control.

*My relationships are a struggle.

*Food makes me sick, unhealthy and fat.

*I am not worth the effort.

*I am unworthy of being fed, nourished and taken care of.

*Food equals comfort.

*Food masks how I really feel.

*Food equals love, feeling loved and being loved.

*I use food to cope with my feelings.

*I use alcohol to cope with my feelings.

*I need to eat a certain way, certain foods, to feel loved; to be loved.

*I eat certain foods to be happy.

*My life is not sweet.

*I punish myself with food.

*I reward myself with food.

*I use food to numb myself and cope with my life.

*I am the fat one, the chubby one, the husky one, the one who struggles with weight.

*I am always the heaviest person in the room.

*Nobody sees me.

*I want to disappear.

*If I lose weight, I will just gain it back and more.

*I am not willing to change anything.

*I want to lose weight without doing anything different.

*I am not willing to step out of my comfort zone.

*I don't love myself or my life.

*I have to hold my tongue and keep quiet.

*I have so much past trauma that I cannot deal with and don't want to deal with.

*My body is sluggish.

*My digestion is sluggish.

*My thyroid is sluggish.

*My emotions are all over the place.

*My hormones are out of whack.

*My lymphatic system is sluggish.

*I am being punished.

*God hates me.

*My family hates me.

*I hate me.

*I have too many toxins in my body.

*I just don't see how I can lose weight.

*It just seems too hard.

*My cells are sluggish.

*Life sucks.

*I blame others for my life.

*Obesity runs in my family.

*If I lose weight my partner will leave me, my friends will hate me and I will be all alone.

*If I lose weight I will leave my partner.

*No one thinks I can lose weight, and I believe them.

*I am weak.

*I am too old to lose weight.

*I have no willpower.

*I need more willpower.

*Willpower is the only way I will lose weight.

*I am a failure.

*I am wrong.

*I hate this planet.

*I don't want to be here.

*People let me down.

*I let myself down.

*I eat because I am bored, tired, sad, lazy, given up on myself.

*I have to do everything and I am exhausted.

*I have no control.

*I am out of control.

*I am not ready to lose weight.

*I am a victim in my life.

*I am a martyr in my life.

*I always sabotage myself.

*I don't make time for myself and my needs.

*I don't know where to begin.

*I am so confused.

*I wish things were different.

*I am hiding behind my excuses.

*I am hiding.

*I think about, obsess over, worry about my weight, wish things were different, hope things will change, want things to change.

*Change is hard.

*Success scares me.

*Failure scares me.

*I feel depressed, anxious, sad and hopeless.

*I feel deprived.

*I am afraid of feeling deprived.

*I am acting rebellious.

*No one is going to tell me what to do.

*Eating is the only joy in my life.

*Eating is the only thing I have control over.

*Other people have told me I am not good enough, and I believed them.

*I have to starve myself to be thinner.

*I have to deprive myself to lose weight.

*I am pissed off about my body and my weight.

*I hate having my picture taken.

*Sugar is my comfort.

*Without sugar I am empty.

*Without sugar I will fall a part.

*People let me down.

*I have let myself down.

*I have to hide my body in baggy, unflattering clothes.

*My body is so flabby.

*I have too much cellulite, so many stretch marks.

*I never reach my goals, so why bother.

*I always fail.

*Something is very wrong with me.

*I can never keep the weight off after I lose it.

*I am just so tired of this struggle.

*Pulling all oaths, vows, contracts, pacts, agreements, curses, hexes to be over-weight in this life; to struggle with weight.

*I feel like I have to clean my plate, otherwise I am being wasteful.

*I need dessert everyday.

*I need a drink at the end of my day to relax, de-stress, numb out, deal with my day.

*I work in a job that I hate.

*My life is not satisfying.

*My relationships are so challenging.

10 ways I can stay focused and motivated!

1.

2.

3.

4.

5.

6.

7.

8.

9.

10.

Reflections so far...

CHAPTER 6

The spiritual causes of being overweight

First and foremost you are a soul in a body, having a human experience. You have lived before this life. You have had so many lifetimes. You have experienced life as different genders, different nationalities, different religious backgrounds, different economic classes, different cultures, so many different times and even on other planets. Whew!

Think about how many issues you have experienced just in this life and then multiply that by a thousand or more lifetimes. Can you fathom how much "stuff", blocked energy, emotional upsets, past traumas you might have running in your subconscious? It can boggle the mind. You can literally carry energy over from other lifetimes that can keep you stuck, slow you down and hold extra weight on your body. Crazy, right? Think about this for a moment and you will see what I mean. Say in another lifetime you were attacked, sexually abused or made to feel like you were too beautiful or too sexy. This in and of itself is horrible. So perhaps in that life you made a vow to yourself or to God that you would never let anything like that happen to you again. Then you come into a new body, in a new lifetime and you have already set yourself for weight struggles.

You may gain weight, so that you are no longer a target for predators or so that you can be invisible and safe. And because of that shock and trauma in that lifetime (or multiple lifetimes) was not truly healed, you bring it into your next lifetime (like invisible suitcases that weigh a ton). And so it goes until the root cause in the root lifetime is healed and integrated. You can bring all sorts of oaths, vows, contracts, pacts, agreements, curses, hexes, etc. into each life that you live until you become aware and do the healing needed to fully let it go.

You can also bring a myriad of trapped emotions, shock, traumas of all kinds, beliefs, basically limiting programming into this life. You can even carry the issues of your ancestors with you from lifetime to lifetime. It is no wonder that you can feel so lost, so stuck, so heavy. You have all this energetic baggage that you are lugging around!

Other spiritual causes of weight struggles include being empathic, which means you pick up other people's emotions and hang onto them as if they are your own. It is like you are a psychic sponge grabbing onto energy that isn't even yours. Have you ever walked into a room and just felt that the energy was heavy or that someone has just been in a fight with someone? You can just feel it. That means that you are sensitive to energy. This is not a bad thing by the way. It is a very good thing to be sensitive. It becomes an issue if you are not able to decipher what is your energy and everyone else's. It can overwhelm you, and you can begin to literally put on weight as a form of protection. You don't have to do this. You can strengthen your own energetic boundaries so that you are not affected by the energy of others. Let me tell you this right now, you are not responsible for anyone's energy. It is not your job to fix or heal or make things better for anyone but yourself. That is your job. Takes the pressure off doesn't it?

Knowing that you are truly only responsible for your body, your thoughts, your actions and reactions, and the happiness and well-being of yourself can be a huge relief. It can be scary too, because now there is no one to blame for your life because you have created it all for yourself (unconsciously most of the time based on beliefs and programming).

Sure people can assist you, guide you, send healing to you, help you heal yourself, show you a new perspective, be a mirror for your own stuff (this happens a lot), but ultimately it is up to you to make the choices that are in alignment with you and your goals.

I love that I am the powerful creator in my own life, and that I can choose to make any changes to my body, my thoughts, beliefs, my health, my life that I desire. And so can you!!

△△△

Quick grounding and protection exercise
to start your day off right!

In order to be fully present in this now moment, I feel it is important to be grounded (to Mother Earth), connected to God (Source, Creator, the Universe) and in my body (aligned and protected). I have a quick exercise that I would love to share with you.

First imagine that you have a grounding cord (it can look like anything you want) that comes down from the base of your spine and anchors deep into the heart of Gaia (Mother Earth). You can also imagine that you have roots coming from the bottom of your feet as well. Make it a visual that pleases you, as there is no wrong way to ground. Your intention to do so is enough.

Then imagine there is a cord moving up your body, through the top of your head that goes up, up, up as high as you can imagine and it plugs into all that is (God, Creator, the Universe, Source). Now set the intention that this Source healing energy runs down your body, filling you with beautiful, healing light energy, clearing away anything that is not of the highest and best love, light and joy. Imagine (and intend) that all of your cells, your organs, your systems, your chakras, your meridians, and your energy bodies are cleansed, cleared, strengthened and aligned. By this time you will be feeling pretty darn good.

If you want to feel a bit more protected, energy wise, you can call upon AA Michael to repair your auric field, and you can even ask that a bubble of white light surrounds you. I do not always do that because I choose to feel safe all the time, but if you have struggled with taking on other people's stuff, you may want to give this a try and see how you feel.

And once this is done, you can just go about your day. Once you practice this a few times, you can literally do this exercise in less than 5 minutes. I sometimes will do this in the shower or when I am driving. Find a time that works for you and just do it. You will feel better if you do. I have recorded this process for you if you prefer to listen. You can find it over at: www.carolinenixon.net/healthy-visualization.html.

Higher Self/Soul Contract

Hello beautiful Spirit, this is your body. In an effort to work together in a way that is pleasurable for us both, I have decided to write a contract for us.

Your soul shines with great light and healing love. Me as the body can sometimes have a hard time processing and grounding it all. Let's work together.

Here is what I propose:

*Daily check ins so that you can tell me what you need.

*Daily grounding by sending my energy down into Mother Earth and connecting to Source by sending my energy up.

*Daily check in of what is ours to do, any guidance we need to hear for our highest and best good.

*Allowing time and patience for me (your body) to catch up with all you are doing and intending.

*Let's build a better and stronger line of communication so that we are in sync.

*Let's also play and lighten up more.

*Show me my gifts and help me develop them.

*Guide me on inspired actions to take that are in alignment for me.

*I propose all of this or something better in our highest and best good.

Name   Date

CHAPTER 7

How you can begin to love your body more

One of the first things you can do, right now, today, is to decide to love yourself. Sounds silly and a bit naive, but the act of claiming it is an important first step in loving yourself and your body more. Do not skip this important step. Also be sure to read through and fill out the body contract (at the end of this chapter). That is a great way to commit to yourself and your happiness.

The body part exercise at the end of chapter 1 is another wonderful way to get into the energy of appreciation, which leads to gratitude and then love, love, love. Sometimes when you can break it down to body parts (ie arms, hips, nose) it is easier to get into the energy of appreciation. Just promise me that you will at least give it a try. You never know what resonates for you if you don't at least try, right?

Another exercise I recommend and have been doing is filling up a "gratitude jar" each day. I use a big, glass mason jar, and each evening before I go to bed, I write down one thing I am grateful for that day. I date it as well, so that at the end of the year I can open up the jar and read through all of the things I was grateful for throughout the year. This is a great family activity as well. We all have so much to be grateful for.

One of my most favorite things to do as a daily/weekly/monthly/ yearly practice is to decide how I want to feel. Let's do this together, so you can see how easy it can be to shift your energy. How do you want to feel in your body? Close your eyes. Take a breath, and allow yourself a moment to come up with a really great feeling word (confident, sexy, peaceful, comfortable, loving, etc). Got how you want to feel? Cool. So, what can you do right now, today to help you feel that way? What tiny little step can you take? Don't wait until you have reached your weight loss goal to feel sexy or confident. Do something, anything to get into that energy right now!

While you are setting your intention on how you want to feel, one of the most powerful exercises you can do right now, today is to begin imagining or visualizing yourself reaching your weight loss goal. I have recorded this exercise for you over at www.caroline-nixon.net so that you can just relax and follow my prompts.

You can also just close your eyes and imagine that there is a full length mirror in front of you. And as you are looking at yourself in this mirror, it shimmers a bit and the new you that you are becoming, the one who has already released the extra body weight, is now staring back at you. Take some time and talk with this new you. Notice what she/he looks like, how happy she/he is. Ask her/him how the goal was reached. Ask her/him for any guidance or support you need to hear.

Allowing yourself to visualize this new you (daily, hourly even) goes a long way to begin reprogramming your subconscious mind. Remember your subconscious mind does not know the difference between what is real and what is made up. When you can imagine/visualize and affirm that this is your new body, your subconscious mind follows along and your body goes along with it, thereby helping you physically achieve your weight loss goal. Athletes do this type of visualizing all the time with great success.

You can also do a self love meditation to get you into the energy of appreciation and love for yourself. Spending just a bit of time daily in gratitude for your body can be so beneficial to raise your overall vibration, get into the energy of love and begin making lasting, positive changes to your body. If you are interested, I have recorded one for you over at www.carolinenixon.net (under the "shop" button).

Reflections so far...

Body Contract

Hello beautiful body, this is your Higher self! As my most cherished employee, I have some new policies and procedures for you to follow, effective immediately. Your incentive package has been upgraded as a result of your excellent performance and the new job requirements.

We are in co-creation in this life, so let's work as a team and have a great time.

As the boss, the new expectations are as follows:

*My body will now and ever more run efficiently, using every single thing eaten as fuel to be burned with the ease of a well oiled machine.

*My body is now very strong and flexible.

*My cells, tissues, organs, muscles, tendons, glands, ligaments, joints and everything else are fully nourished, satisfied & well lubricated.

*My body now has tons of energy, all day long.

*I am able to move my body with ease, grace and perfect alignment.

*My body will inform me when it needs something, and I will make sure that the needs are met in a timely manner.

*My mood is now even, calm, neutral and full of happiness and joy.

*My body releases any extra body weight that it has been holding onto for whatever reason, cause, block with ease, grace and perfect alignment.

*My body is now grounded to Mother Earth and connected to Source (Creator) at all times.

*My body and energy field are surrounded by golden, white light and is protected at all times.

*All of my body's needs, wants and desires are now met (and exceeded).

*My body is 100% healthy, vibrant and youthful.

Incentive package includes but is not limited to:

*We get to enjoy at least one week of vacation each calendar year.

*Self care as needed/desired including massages, writing, reading, napping, quiet time, exercise, eating delicious foods, having adventures, spending time with those I love, etc.

As the boss, I promise to talk to you with love and compassion from this day forward. I forgive myself for being so hard on myself. I will coach/mentor you so that you know how much I appreciate you.

Name   Date

10 things about my body that I am grateful for!

1.

2.

3.

4.

5.

6.

7.

8.

9.

10.

"Courage doesn't always roar. Sometimes courage is the little voice at the end of the day that says I'll try again tomorrow."

-Mary Anne Radmacher

CHAPTER 8

How you can begin to release your "stuff"

This chapter is going to help you continue to release all those limiting, low vibin beliefs, thoughts and programming that are keeping you from reaching your goal of your most healthy weight and loving yourself so much more. At the end of chapter 5 there was a very extensive list of limiting beliefs that I have found to be so common with my clients and their inability to release weight. These beliefs just hang out in the subconscious mind and run the show in your life.

Even if you consciously think that you want to lose weight, and that this time is going to be different, after a bit of time those pesky limiting, un-truths that are anchored into the subconscious mind begin to surface and they begin to wreak havoc in your efforts to lose weight. And the cycle continues over and over again until those beliefs can be addressed, pulled and reprogrammed. I will be sharing a very long list of new, higher vibin, positive belief statements that you can use to reprogram your subconscious mind to more self love and easier weight loss at the end of this chapter.

So what can you do to reprogram your subconscious mind so that you can love yourself more and release more weight with ease? You can journal. Writing down your limiting beliefs (see chapter 5 for some ideas), and really getting into them, exploring where they are present in your life is a great exercise.

You can get energy healing to help identify and pull your limiting, un-truths while unblocking your energy, so that you body can move into more balance and harmony (which helps you lose weight).

Hypnosis is another tool you can use to lose weight. Hypnosis reprograms the subconscious mind for all kinds of issues; not just weight.

Meditation can help you become more mindful of your body, your thoughts, and it can bring great peace to your life. Simply sitting with your hands on your heart and taking slow, deep breaths can be sooooo good for you and your peace of mind.

You can also begin working with your Higher self and your spirit guide team (those angels, teachers sand masters who help you in this life). I have created a powerful meditation where I help you call in your very own "weight loss" spirit guide. Having a spirit guide that directly supports your self love and weight loss efforts can be so beneficial to your success. You can find it over at www. caroline.net.

You can work with affirmations and afformations as well. I go into these more over in chapter 9, so do be sure to check that out.

These are but a few of the many ways you can begin to shift your focus towards your true desires of more self love and easier weight loss. Do be sure to set the intention as well. The simple act of just setting the intention for health, self love and weight loss is like a beacon to the Universe that you are ready for all the good stuff and the support from Source, God, the Universe.

All you need to do to set your intention is repeat the statement I have created for you (although you can change the words if you like).

"I (state your name) now set the intention for so much more self love, love of my body, health in all parts of my body, mind and soul, AND I set the intention that my body will rebalance itself to my most perfect and healthy weight. In my highest and best good I send this intention out into the Universe and I request that my spirit team, my Higher self and all aspects of me help me, guide me and support me, now and always. Thank you. And so it is."

△△△

Body, body, body exercise

Sometimes we look outside ourselves for the answers we seek for our life. We ask our friends what they think we should do, our partners, our family, psychics, healers, therapists, everyone but the one person who actually knows you and your body best.

You! You have all the knowledge and wisdom within you. You just need to tune in. Do you know how to tap into all of that? It is not that hard to do when you decide to stop going outside of yourself and turn your attention and intention inward.

Try this daily practice. Ask your body this question, "Body, body, body, what do you need today to be the healthiest and happiest body possible?" Or you can ask, "Body, body, body, what do you need to begin releasing weight?" Then listen. You will hear, see, get a sense of, know the exact thing your body needs in that moment. The voice may whisper that you need water, rest, more fun, or you will get a feeling of something you could do. You may see it in your mind's eye.

Honor what you receive and thank your body for telling you. The more you play with this exercise, the louder the inner voice will be and the more confident you will feel with this new skill. You are building a connection with your amazing body.

When you make the time to listen to what your body needs everyday, your body doesn't have to become sick or dis-eased to grab your attention. Once your body has physical symptoms of disharmony, I promise you that your body has been trying to get your attention for a long time.

This quick exercise will also help you to trust your inner wisdom the more you tune in (do it at least daily if not more). This act of self love tells your body that you love it so much that you want to know what it needs. Promise yourself to at least give this easy exercise a try for a week. The more you do it, the easier it will be and the more information you will begin to receive as well. And your intuitive senses will become more heightened, so bonus.

Journal Time

I overeat and/or eat less healthy foods because?

____

____

____

____

____

____

____

How are your relationships with your partner, family and friends?

____

____

____

____

"If you think you can do a
thing or think can can't do
a thing, you're right."

-Henry Ford

Positive beliefs to bring into your body, mind & soul

Below are a lot of new and improved, positive belief statements that you can use to replace all of the limiting ones in your subconscious mind (think upgrading your internal hard drive). You can use these like you would an affirmation, or you can head over to my website at www.carolinenixon.net and check out the energy healing recording bundle I made for you.

*I know why my body is holding onto extra weight.

*I know what I need to do to begin to release my extra weight.

*I know what my body needs to feel great and be healthy.

*My body knows what to do.

*My mind knows what to do.

*My soul knows what to do.

*My mind is on board with making new choices.

*All foods are friendly to me and my body.

*I am motivated and guided daily.

*I allow it to be easy for me to lose weight.

*I give myself permission to love my body.

*I give myself permission to release weight easily.

*I am confident in my body's ability to release weight with ease and grace.

*I am confident.

*I know what it feels like to easily release weight.

*I know what it feels like to love all foods.

*I know what it feels like to be nourished by the foods I eat.

*I know what it feels like to enjoy eating.

*I know what it feels like to let go of my strict dieting beliefs.

*I know how to allow more love into my life.

*I know what it feels like to love myself fully.

*I know how to let go of control.

*I know how to allow more flow and ease into my life.

*I know what it feels like to nourish myself in healthy ways.

*Eating is safe for me.

*My life is sweet.

*I love my food, and my food loves me.

*I know what it feels like to be comforted without using food.

*I enjoy what I eat, and my food nourishes me.

*I feel satisfied and fulfilled.

*I feel sexy.

*I am so worthy of all the sweetness in life.

*I know what it feels like to be loved without using sugar, or any other food.

*I know what it feels like to live without using food to love myself, to comfort myself, to console myself or to mask my feelings.

*I know how to listen to my body and give it what it needs.

*I know how to live my life without anger, guilt, shame and/or resentment.

*I know how to express my feelings in healthy ways.

*I know how to let go of past hurts that are affecting my health and my weight.

*I know what being healthy feels like.

*I know what being at my perfect weight feels like.

*I know what being beautiful feels like.

*I am safe.

*I am secure.

*I am grounded.

*It is safe to be in my body.

*It is safe to be visible; to be seen.

*It is safe to be beautiful.

*I know what it feels like to be slimmer and safe, respected, grounded, happy, be loved and get my needs met.

*I know what it feels like to love myself no matter what the scale says.

*I know what it feels like to love myself no matter how much I weigh and what size I am.

*I am worth loving.

*I know what it feels like to move my body in ways that feel good.

*It is fun for me to move my body daily.

*I am worth the effort.

*My body craves movement daily.

*It is easy for me to move my body in healthy ways.

*Exercise is actually fun for me.

*My body knows exactly how and when to move and groove and it feels so good.

*I love moving my body.

*Every movement I make builds strength in my body.

*I love my body and my body loves me.

*I know what it feels like to be excited and passionate.

*I know what it feels like to have tons of energy, all day long.

*I know what it feels like to love who I see in the mirror.

*I know what it feels like to be grateful for my body.

*I know what it feels like to let go of my extra weight with ease.

*I know what it feels like to live without being overweight; without struggling with my weight.

*I know how to heal my body's metabolism.

*I know what it feels like to have great metabolism.

*I know what it feels like to have balanced hormones.

*I know what it feels like to be the perfect weight for me.

*I know what it feels like to have a balanced relationship with all foods.

*I am at peace with myself.

*I am at peace with my feelings.

*I am at peace with my body.

*I deserve the best.

*I am willing and do forgive myself and my past actions.

*I forgive myself for berating my body for so very long.

*I love my body.

*I love my organs.

*I love all of my flaws, my scars, my stretch marks, my cellulite, my veins, my muffin top, my saddle bags, moles, freckles, birthmarks. I love all of me!

*I am strong.

*I know what it feels like to have wonderful, nurturing relationships.

*I know what it feels like to be supported.

*I forgive myself for how I have treated my body in the past.

*I know how to release anger, hatred, resentment, guilt and shame in healthy ways.

*I know what it feels like to be worthy of the best.

*I know what deep healing feels like.

*I know what it feels like to live in balance and harmony with my body, my emotions; all things.

*My ego easily gets on board with my desire to release weight.

*I know how to live in joy, peace, balance and harmony.

*I know what it feels like to be happy.

*My inner child happily and joyfully helps me to release weight.

*My ego feels safe while I am releasing weight.

*I know what unconditional love feels like.

*I know what it feels like to happily have pictures taken of me.

*I know how to forgive my parents, grandparents, adoptive parents, caregivers, siblings and myself for any past hurts/experiences.

*I know what it feels like to be comfortable in my body and in my own skin.

*I know how to accept changes in my life without inner resistance.

I know how to identify what emotions are mine, and what emotions belong to other people, and I am easily able to release what is not mine.

*I am protected and I know what it feels like to be protected.

*I know what it feels like to have excellent boundaries.

*I know how to say "no" and not feel guilty.

*I know what it feels like to confidently uphold strong boundaries.

*I enjoy eating slowly.

*I know what being successful feels like.

*I know what reaching a goal feels like.

"With everything that has happened to you, you can either feel sorry for yourself or treat what has happened as a gift. Everything is either an opportunity to grow or an obstacle to keep you from growing. You get to choose."

-D. Wayne Dyer

CHAPTER 9

Cool tools to help you release weight

In this chapter, you will learn tons of tips, tricks, hacks, short cuts, whatever you want to call them to help you release weight with more ease and joy (yes, joy). I am including some of my most favorite things here; stuff that has worked for me (and my clients). Do not feel like you have to use all of these tools. Be open. Try one on and see how it fits for you. If it doesn't resonate, that is totally fine. Move onto the next one.

First off, let's talk about Aromatherapy. I have been a certified Aromatherapist for about 20 years. To say I love essential oils is an understatement. Aromatherapy is easy, fun and powerful (it's a triple threat). So what is Aromatherapy and how do you use it to help with weight struggles? By definition, Aromatherapy is a branch of Herbology which uses highly concentrated pure essential oils that are distilled from plants, flowers, shrubs and trees. Aromatherapy is used to restore or enhance all aspects of health, beauty and overall well-being.

Aromatherapy has been around a very long time. Ancient burial sites as far back at 80,000 BC showed signs of the use of plants, flowers and elixirs. Ayurvedic medicine in India was born around 4800 BC and used herbs, flowers and plants for healing. Even the Bible has references of the use of plants (Frankincense, Myrrh, Spikenard).

More recently in the 1920's, the term Aromatherapy was coined by a French chemist named Rene Maurice Gettefosse. In the 1940's Dr. Jean Valnet used essential oils to heal wounds on the battlefield during World War II. Several countries in Europe have regularly used essential oils since the 1950's in their healing practices and in some hospitals.

As you can see, the art of Aromatherapy is not some hippy-dippy, new age nonsense. It has been scientifically studied and successfully practiced all over the world for an extremely long time.

Now that the history lesson is over, let's get to the fun stuff. I want to briefly go over what to look for when you go to the store and buy your essential oils and how to use them once you bring them home. I have included a chart to share which oils specifically are great as weight loss supporters. Know that essential oils are so multifaceted though, with amazing healing properties for the mind, body and soul.

When you are looking to buy essential oils, it is important to keep a few things in mind. First off, look for oils that are 100% pure (as in no other ingredients). The label will say what is in the bottle. You don't want any fillers in your oils. There are a lot of essential oil companies that have some pretty impressive sales tactics, but don't be fooled. Organic oils are great if you can afford them. I use a lot of oils that are not organic with great success though. Also you want to make sure the full plant name is on the bottle, so that you know which plant type you are purchasing. There are several types of Lavender for instance. I only buy from companies where I know what is in my bottle, where it was grown and that there are no impurities in the finished product.

Some oils which are expensive are the only exception to this rule as they will be 10% of the essential oil and 90% jojoba (or another carrier oil). Rose is a great example of this. Rose essential is ridiculously pricey, so I will buy it in a carrier oil.

Next you want to purchase oils that are only in dark bottles (glass). Essential oils are affected by heat and light, so it is important that they be kept in dark bottles (amber or cobalt are the most common) and out of the heat.

Finally if you see a line of essential oils that are all the same price, you might want to keep looking. Lavender essential oil is way cheaper than Rose essential oil. It is about the process of making the oil, how much plant matter is needed, where the plants come from, etc. that determines the price.

Once you have selected your essential oils, now what? The easiest way to use essential oils is to open up the bottle and take a big whiff. Seriously, it is that simple. When you smell an essential oil, the molecules travel up the nasal cavity and into the limbic system of your brain (your old brain; the memory center). So smelling the oil this way is the best and fastest way to receive the benefits for your body, mind and soul.

There are some folks (and companies) that tell you to put the oils on the bottom of your feet, rub the oils on your spine, drink or cook with the oils, and a bunch of other applications. For the most part I do not advocate any of these methods. I don't think they are particularly safe for some people, and in truth they just are not needed. Open the bottle and smell the oil; boom, you are done. You can add essential oils to a massage oil however with great success, especially for muscle aches and increasing circulation to help with cellulite. And using a diffuser in a large room is a great way to purify the air and permeate a big space with aromas. I have several diffusers in my home. If you have pets though, do your research as essential oils can actually have a negative effect on your fur babies (especially cats).

Personally, I love making Aromatherapy inhalers using essential oils. An inhaler is a plastic tube (or metal) that has a cotton insert that you put a few drops of essential oil on, close it up, then you unscrew the top to smell your oils. I love them because you can carry them with you without worrying about spilling your precious essential oils. You can look these up online. They come in tons of colors (I love using color to enhance the intention of the oils) and they are pretty cheap. Do be sure to research what oils you use as some can have contraindications for certain health issues and medications. Generally speaking essential oils are super safe, effective and smell amazing.

Essential Oils for Releasing Weight

Essential oils are a powerful tool you can use to assist with releasing weight, raising your vibes, clearing your mind and keeping you motivated. Below is a list of a few of my favorites for releasing weight. Remember to always consult with an Aromatherapist before using essential oils. Some oils have contraindications like pregnancy, epilepsy, certain cancers, etc.

*Cinnamon: can help with digestion and increasing metabolism

*Fennel: can help with fluid retention

*Ginger: can help with digestion

*Grapefruit: can help detox the body

*Juniper: can help with bloating

*Lemon: can help detox and energize the body

*Orange: can help elevate the mood

*Peppermint: can help with digestion

*Rosemary: can help reduce cellulite

△△△

The next cool tool I want to talk with you about is crystals. Yes crystals. No they are not just rocks. They are powerful, vibrational healers. The reason I love using crystals in my healing practice is because not only are they beautiful to look at, but they literally raise your vibration and help you release your "stuff" when you work with them. Remember that everything is energy and has a unique frequency. Crystals are pure, high vibin and they lift you up to meet their vibration. There are countless books available on crystals, so if these little gems call to you, by all means research away.

The one thing that I do want to spend a minute talking about it what to do once you bring a new crystal home. Nowadays you can buy crystals online and in new age type shops. There are cheaper fake or man-made crystals available, so it is important to buy from a reputable store and not at the gas station.

It is super important to cleanse your crystals when you bring them home. You can do this a number of ways. My favorite way is to use a sage bundle and allow the smoke to cleanse the crystal. Some crystals can be placed in soapy water, some can be buried in dirt or rice. You can put your crystals out in the moonlight to get cleansed and recharged. You can use sound, breath or even just your intention to cleanse your stones. There are many ways to cleanse them. Again, I find using sage to be the quickest and easiest, but you can play with a few and see which ones you enjoy the most. Do an internet search as well for more information. Softer crystals need to be handled differently than a harder type.

Once your crystals are cleansed, you might want to consider giving them a job. Yes, give your crystals something to do for you. It is called programming. It is not too difficult to do at all. What I do is pick the stone I want to work with, make sure it has been cleansed (I use sage and intention), then I hold the crystal in my hands as I speak the intention I have for it. If releasing weight is your intention (which I am assuming it is since you are reading this book), simply choose a crystal (see the list below) that resonates for you, and say something like, "This crystal that I am holding (you can name it) is going to help me ....(reduce cravings, speed up my metabolism, love my body more, etc) every time I hold it or look at it. Thank you. It is done." It can really be that simple.

Now you need to follow through and actually hold the crystal, meditate with it, gaze at it, make a crystal grid, etc. You cannot just set the intention then forget all about the crystal. It won't work for you if you do that.

I like to keep small polished stones in my car, so that I can pick one up as I am driving. They can be a great reminder of your goals, they can motivate you, help you with a food craving, calm you down, heal your body. Play with these magical beauties and see what happens for you.

Crystals for Releasing Weight

Crystals are a powerful tool to help you release weight. Simply holding the crystal, meditating with or gazing at the crystal can bring so much balance and healing.

*Amethyst: can help in reducing cravings and letting go of emotions

*Apatite: can help decrease your appetite while increasing metabolism; it can also turn fear into action

*Blue Lace Agate: can help you say no to unhealthy foods

*Carnelian: can help give you an energy boost and have more fun

*Citrine: can help with digestion, metabolism, intentions and confidence

*Goldstone: can help you stick to your goals

*Green Opal: can help you promote healthy dietary habits

*Iolite: can help you release fatty deposits

*Kunzite: can help you love your body more

*Ocean Jasper: can help stimulate body movements

*Malachite: can help with making conscious choices and taking more confident actions

*Rose Quartz: can help you have compassion and love for yourself and your body

*Red Tiger's Eye: can help increase metabolism

*Sodalite: can help it all be easier

*Sunstone: can help decrease the appetite while increasing the metabolism

*Topaz: can help with setting intentions and having clear boundaries

*Black Tourmaline: can help you feel safe, release negative energy and ground yourself

△△△

Affirmations can be powerful reminders to keep you motivated on your releasing weight journey. Sometime however I find that affirmations don't work very quickly because we don't actually believe the positive statement that we are saying. I do think it is beneficial though to be surrounded with positive affirmations. The following are not only positive intention statements (or affirmations), but they are also energetic feeling downloads. I have set the intention that everyone who reads these statements will be "downloaded" or given energy healing (yes you can do this-everything is just energy). Trust that as you read the statements, the positive energy from them is swirling around you and into your very core. Feel free to make your own affirmations that light you up. You can write them on sticky pads and put them all over your home, you can record yourself reading them, you can use them as a screensaver for your phone, and you can program your crystals with an affirmation so that each time you pick

up and hold your crystal, the affirmation comes through and reminds you.

*I know what it feels like to be confident in my body.

*I know what it feels like to be healthy.

*I know what it feels like to make good food choices that I love.

*I know what it feels like to move my body daily in ways that feel
great.

*I know what it feels like to make time for myself everyday.

*I know what it feels like to really enjoy myself; to have fun.

*I know what it feels like to release weight and feel great.

*I know what it feels like to have healthy boundaries.

*I know what it feels like to release weight easily.

*I know what it feels like to be proud of myself.

*I know what it feels like to reach my weight loss goals.

*I know what it feels like to get my needs met.

*I know what it feels like to trust myself.

*I know what it feels like to take action.

*I know what it feels like to be safe in my body and on this planet.

*I know what it feels like to fully relax and let go.

*I know what it feels like to love all me, including my body.

*I know what it feels like to trust my intuition.

*I know what it feels like to be happy.

*My body runs like a well oiled machine.

*I know what it feels like to be totally, freaking awesome!!

△△△

As affirmations are positive intention statements, afformations are positive intention questions. You see, your mind is curious by nature and loves, loves, loves to answer questions. When you state something as a positive question, your mind begins to look for ways to answer the question. I cannot take credit for coming up with this amazing tool, but I do use afformations a lot. Check out "The stuff to check out" section at the end of this book for more information on afformations. Below are some great affor-mations to get you started. I like to ask myself these questions all throughout my day. It is really cool if you find yourself being mean and bullying your body, to recognize that you are doing that, stop and then ask yourself one of these afformations. It can flip the switch on negative self talk.

*Why am I so healthy?

*Why am I confident?

*Why is my body releasing weight so easily?

*Why am I taking such good care of myself?

*Why do I love myself so much?

*Why do I always have so much fun?

*Why is my life so amazing?

*Why are my relationships so amazing?

*Why is it so easy for me to reach my weight loss goals?

*Why am I so amazing?

*Why am I so fulfilled?

*Why am I so joyful?

*Why am I so happy, healthy and wealthy?

Journal Time

What do you love most about yourself?

Where are you holding yourself back in your life?

Why are you resisting making new changes in your life?

What are your biggest fears about NOT releasing weight?

Where can you forgive yourself?

____

____

____

____

____

____

Quick tip if you have a craving

If you find yourself craving something that you know is not super nourishing or healthy and you really don't want to eat it, try this exercise. Remember that I said that it is okay to eat anything as long as you eat it with total love and appreciation while you bless the heck out of it? If you eat something and feel guilt or shame afterwards, you have just ingested a bunch of guilt and shame.

Let's say you just want to get rid of the craving though. All you need to do is stop what you are doing and take a slow, deep, cleansing breath. Then take another deep breath. If you are using essential oils and/or crystals, now is the time to bring them out. Hold the crystal and smell the oil to bring yourself back into this now moment.

Ask your body what it really needs right now. It may be that you just need a glass of water or a hug (seriously). If that craving is still happening, you can say "DELETE" out loud (unless you are in a store and people are all around you). Saying "delete" out loud can help disrupt the energy around the craving.

You can also do this if you catch yourself being mean to yourself with negative self talk. Interrupt the negativity by saying "No or delete". You can also visualize a big, red rubber stamp that reads "no, complete or delete" as those negative thoughts come up. See the rubber stamp literally stamping out those thoughts like they would on a piece of paper. Get into it. Imagine or visualize it as much as you can. It really works. Give it a try and see for yourself.

But remember if you really want that thing you are craving, by all means enjoy it with 100% of your being. If you demonize foods, they will demonize and control you. Be at peace with all foods and you will be at peace. I have created a quick energy healing recording that you can use anytime you get a craving that you would prefer to not indulge in. Check it out over at www.caroline.net.

WEEKLY CHECKLIST OF POSITIVE ACTIONS FOR BETTER HEALTH AND WEIGHT RELEASING

	MONDAY	TUESDAY	WEDNESDAY	THURSDAY	FRIDAY	SATURDAY	SUNDAY
I WROTE IN MY JOURNAL TODAY.							
I MOVED MY BODY TODAY.							
I ADDED A VEGETABLE/FRUIT TO MY DIET TODAY.							
I STAYED HYDRATED TODAY.							
I SPENT SOME TIME IN NATURE TODAY.							
I CHECKED IN WITH MY BODY TODAY.							
I WAS KIND WITH MYSELF TODAY.							

MONTHLY EXERCISE LOG

If you are a visual person, feel free to use this simple chart
to keep track of your exercise throughout the month.

MONDAY	TUESDAY	WEDNESDAY	THURSDAY	FRIDAY	SATURDAY	SUNDAY

Celebrate your success!

What new actions, thoughts, beliefs, habits, successes can you celebrate this week, this month, this year??

What have you learned about yourself by reading this book?

____

____

____

Setting your weight loss goal

1. What is your weight loss goal (be specific)?

2. How will you feel once you have reached your goal?

3. Why do you want to lose weight (your big reasons)?

4. What is your timeline for reaching your goal?

5. What action can you take right now to get into the feeling you stated in question #2?

6. Check in with yourself daily.

7. Take more actions.

8. Reassess often if what you are doing is getting you the results you want? If not, course correct.

9. Spend a few moments daily visualizing yourself reaching your weight loss goal.

Monthly Menu Plan

For years I have used a monthly dinner menu chart like the one below. It takes me very little time to fill this chart out, and then I am able to quickly throw together a shopping list for the week and move onto other things. I am the kind of gal that needs to have a menu plan for the week, otherwise I will order too much take out. Feel free to use this template or create your own. I post my menu plan on the refrigerator, so that everyone knows what is for dinner.

MONDAY	TUESDAY	WEDNESDAY	THURSDAY	FRIDAY	SATURDAY	SUNDAY

Your body as a pendulum

You can use your body's wisdom to find out if something you eat (or if a supplement) is good for your body by using your body as a pendulum. This "yes/no" technique will help you to easily receive your body's inner knowing. Begin by standing up and taking some deep breaths and letting go of any expectation (super important). Just be open to receive the answer in your highest and best good.

*Decide what a "Yes" answer feels like (perhaps your body sways forwards).

*Decide what a "No" answer feels like (maybe your body sways backwards).

*Take a deep breath while letting go of any expectations.

*Set the intention to receive the answer in your highest good.

*Practice with simple Yes/No questions (like your name).

*Once you have practiced and have begun to build trust in your body and your ability to receive answers, begin testing the foods, supplements, vitamins that you want.

*The more you practice, the easier this technique will feel and the more you will trust your body's wisdom.

*If you feel like you are getting weird answers, stop practicing, clear your energy (by drinking some water and taking some breaths) and begin again.

Remember that letting go of your expectations is important with this. Play with this exercise. It can prove to be super valuable if you are standing in a store with a million supplement choices and no idea which one to purchase.

Final reflections...

STUFF TO CHECK OUT

Here are a few of my all time favorite authors, books and products. They are in no particular order.

Donna Eden-anything by her is amazing!

The Book of Afformations by Noah St. John

Essential Aromatherapy, a pocket guide to essential oils and Aromatherapy by Susan Worwood (Anything by her is awesome though.)

The Crystal Healer by Philip Permutt is a great book if you like pictures of crystals.

Dr. Joe Dispenza-his work is fantastic.

Judy Hall-her books on crystals are great.

Louise Hay-was a pioneer in using affirmations for healing.

The National Association for Holistic Aromatherapy is a great resource. www.naha.org

Atlantic Institute of Aromatherapy is another awesome resource. www.atlanticinstitute.com.

If you are looking for natural cleaning solutions, check out the company Norwex. I am not an affiliate, but I love their stuff. The cleaning cloths are amazing.

For natural makeup options, check out www.Beautycounter.com. I am not an affiliate, but I really like their products.

EPILOGUE

It has been such a pleasure sharing all that I know, have studied and my experiences with my own weight struggles and body image issues. I, like you, are a work in progress. I learn and grow every single day. By the time this book is printed, I will have thought of more information, more exercises, more journal entry prompts to give you in order to help you heal your relationship with yourself and your body.

As a recovering perfectionist however, sometimes you just have to hit "publish" and let it be. So if you like what you have read, and you want to learn more, I humbly invite you to check out my website (www.carolinenixon.net), get on my emailing list or come over to Facebook and say hello.

I am so proud of you for daring to dig deeper into your beliefs and internal programming. I can tell you that not too many folks want to do this internal work. They would rather keep on the dieting roller coaster and silently berating themselves for not succeeding. You are amazing. You are unique and divine, and I know that you can be successful at any goal you set for yourself.

You have a lot of tools in your tool-belt to assist you on your journey.

It has been my honor to shine a light on your path. Please reach out and let me know how you are doing and how I can support you further. Until we meet again, here's to your health and wellness.

BOOKS BY THIS AUTHOR

A Mom's Guide To Sanity

We moms are all hard workers. Sometimes the sheer monotony of the day with all the various routines is enough to send even the most patient of moms running to the nearest bar or all-you-can eat buffet. This book is full of fast and easy ways to cope with all the craziness and chaos that we have in our lives. This book illustrates very simple and inexpensive techniques you can employ to keep yourself sane. You deserve to lead a healthier, more balanced and spiritual life.

An Itsy, Bitsy, Teeny, Weeny Guide To Life

We so easily look outside ourselves for health advice, relationship advice and everything else in between. We look to doctors, therapists and psychics to tell us what is going on within our own body. While we should seek out professional assistance when we need it, we would do well to listen to the quiet part of ourselves, which is so wise. Within this book holds many fast and easy techniques to help bring you more balance, joy and spirit into your life.

ABOUT THE AUTHOR

Caroline Nixon

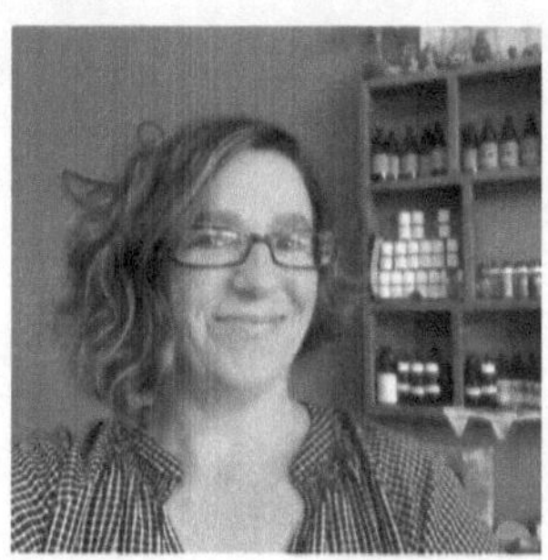 is an absolutely magical healer, teacher and author with an amazing sense of humor to balance out the sacred work she does. Caroline uses her 20 years of experience in all things holistic to help women reclaim their health and lose weight with way more ease, flow and of course joy!! She is also the author of A Mom's Guide to Sanity and An Itsy, Bitsy, Teeny, Weeny Guide to Life.

Her journey in massage therapy, hypnosis, aromatherapy expanding into her Reiki Master level, reading and healing in the Akashic Records and more has helped Caroline discover and release the deep blocks holding her clients back from experiencing total health and vitality. Caroline believes that we are each so very powerful, and we need only step into that power to create anything we choose.

You can find Caroline at:
www.carolinenixon.net
www.facebook.com/thecarolinenixon
www.instagram.com/thecarolinenixon